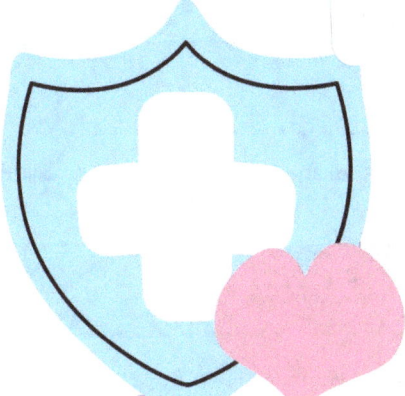

Health-Care meets Self-Care:
The Chronic Illness Details

Name	
Address	
Phone	

© Alana Parisotto, 2023

Table of Contents

Medical Profile

Full Name	
D.O.B.	Blood Type
Allergies	

Diagnosed Condition	Year

Medical Card & Account Details			
Type / Company	Number	Ref	Expiry

Doctors & Specialists

Name		Phone	
Specialty			
Clinic			
Email			
Address			
Notes			

Name		Phone	
Specialty			
Clinic			
Email			
Address			
Notes			

Name		Phone	
Specialty			

Clinic	
Email	
Address	
Notes	

Name		Phone	
Specialty			
Clinic			
Email			
Address			
Notes			

Name		Phone	
Specialty			
Clinic			
Email			
Address			

Notes	

Name		Phone	
Specialty			
Clinic			
Email			
Address			
Notes			

Name		Phone	
Specialty			
Clinic			
Email			
Address			
Notes			

Name		Phone	
Specialty			

Clinic	
Email	
Address	
Notes	

Name		Phone	
Specialty			
Clinic			
Email			
Address			
Notes			

Name		Phone	
Specialty			
Clinic			
Email			
Address			

Notes	

Name		Phone	
Specialty			
Clinic			
Email			
Address			
Notes			

Name		Phone	
Specialty			
Clinic			
Email			
Address			
Notes			

Name		Phone	
Specialty			

Clinic	
Email	
Address	
Notes	

Name		Phone	
Specialty			
Clinic			
Email			
Address			
Notes			

Name		Phone	
Specialty			
Clinic			
Email			
Address			

Notes	

Name		Phone	
Specialty			
Clinic			
Email			
Address			
Notes			

Name		Phone	
Specialty			
Clinic			
Email			
Address			
Notes			

Name		Phone	
Specialty			

Clinic	
Email	
Address	
Notes	

Name		Phone	
Specialty			
Clinic			
Email			
Address			
Notes			

Name		Phone	
Specialty			
Clinic			
Email			
Address			

Notes	

Name		Phone	
Specialty			
Clinic			
Email			
Address			
Notes			

Name		Phone	
Specialty			
Clinic			
Email			
Address			
Notes			

Name		Phone	
Specialty			

Clinic	
Email	
Address	
Notes	

Name		Phone	
Specialty			
Clinic			
Email			
Address			
Notes			

Name		Phone	
Specialty			
Clinic			
Email			
Address			

Notes	

Pharmacies & Chemists

Name	
Phone	
Email	
Address	
Notes	

Name	
Phone	
Email	
Address	
Notes	

Name	

Phone	
Email	
Address	
Notes	

Name	
Phone	
Email	
Address	
Notes	

Name	
Phone	
Email	
Address	
Notes	

Name	
Phone	
Email	
Address	
Notes	

Name	
Phone	
Email	
Address	
Notes	

Name	
Phone	
Email	
Address	

Notes	

Name	
Phone	
Email	
Address	
Notes	

Name	
Phone	
Email	
Address	
Notes	

Name	
Phone	
Email	

Address	
Notes	

Name	
Phone	
Email	
Address	
Notes	

Name	
Phone	
Email	
Address	
Notes	

Name	

Phone	
Email	
Address	
Notes	

Name	
Phone	
Email	
Address	
Notes	

Name	
Phone	
Email	
Address	
Notes	

Symptoms List

Type		Condition	
Location		Regularity	
Start Date		End Date	
Description			

Type		Condition	
Location		Regularity	
Start Date		End Date	
Description			

Type		Condition	
Location		Regularity	
Start Date		End Date	
Description			

Type		Condition	
Location		Regularity	
Start Date		End Date	
Description			

Type		Condition	
Location		Regularity	
Start Date		End Date	
Description			

Type		Condition	
Location		Regularity	
Start Date		End Date	
Description			

Type		Condition	
Location		Regularity	
Start Date		End Date	
Description			

Type		Condition	
Location		Regularity	
Start Date		End Date	
Description			

Type		Condition	
Location		Regularity	
Start Date		End Date	
Description			

Type		Condition	
Location		Regularity	
Start Date		End Date	
Description			

Type		Condition	
Location		Regularity	
Start Date		End Date	
Description			

Type		Condition	
Location		Regularity	
Start Date		End Date	
Description			

Type		Condition	
Location		Regularity	
Start Date		End Date	
Description			

Type		Condition	
Location		Regularity	
Start Date		End Date	
Description			

Type		Condition	
Location		Regularity	
Start Date		End Date	
Description			

Type		Condition	
Location		Regularity	
Start Date		End Date	
Description			

Type		Condition	
Location		Regularity	
Start Date		End Date	
Description			

Type		Condition	
Location		Regularity	
Start Date		End Date	
Description			

Type		Condition	
Location		Regularity	
Start Date		End Date	
Description			

Type		Condition	
Location		Regularity	
Start Date		End Date	
Description			

Type		Condition	
Location		Regularity	
Start Date		End Date	
Description			

Type		Condition	
Location		Regularity	
Start Date		End Date	
Description			

Type		Condition	
Location		Regularity	
Start Date		End Date	
Description			

Type		Condition	
Location		Regularity	
Start Date		End Date	
Description			

Type		Condition	
Location		Regularity	
Start Date		End Date	
Description			

Type		Condition	
Location		Regularity	
Start Date		End Date	
Description			

Type		Condition	
Location		Regularity	
Start Date		End Date	
Description			

Type		Condition	
Location		Regularity	
Start Date		End Date	
Description			

Type		Condition	
Location		Regularity	
Start Date		End Date	
Description			

Type		Condition	
Location		Regularity	
Start Date		End Date	
Description			

Trialed Treatments

Name	Condition	Time Period

& Medications List

Purpose	Outcome

Name	Condition	Time Period

Purpose	Outcome

Name	Condition	Time Period

Purpose	Outcome

Name	Condition	Time Period

Purpose	Outcome

Surgeries & Procedures

When		Doctor	
Condition		Location	
Description			

When		Doctor	
Condition		Location	
Description			

When		Doctor	
Condition		Location	
Description			

When		Doctor	
Condition		Location	
Description			

When		Doctor	

Condition		Location	
Description			

When		Doctor	
Condition		Location	
Description			

When		Doctor	
Condition		Location	
Description			

When		Doctor	
Condition		Location	
Description			

When		Doctor	
Condition		Location	
Description			

When		Doctor	
Condition		Location	
Description			

When		Doctor	
Condition		Location	
Description			

When		Doctor	
Condition		Location	
Description			

When		Doctor	
Condition		Location	
Description			

When		Doctor	
Condition		Location	

Description	

When		Doctor	
Condition		Location	
Description			

When		Doctor	
Condition		Location	
Description			

When		Doctor	
Condition		Location	
Description			

When		Doctor	
Condition		Location	
Description			

When		Doctor	
Condition		Location	
Description			

When		Doctor	
Condition		Location	
Description			

When		Doctor	
Condition		Location	
Description			

When		Doctor	
Condition		Location	
Description			

When		Doctor	
Condition		Location	

Description	

When		Doctor	
Condition		Location	
Description			

When		Doctor	
Condition		Location	
Description			

When		Doctor	
Condition		Location	
Description			

When		Doctor	
Condition		Location	
Description			

When		Doctor	
Condition		Location	
Description			

When		Doctor	
Condition		Location	
Description			

When		Doctor	
Condition		Location	
Description			

When		Doctor	
Condition		Location	
Description			

When		Doctor	
Condition		Location	

Description	

When		Doctor	
Condition		Location	

Description	

When		Doctor	
Condition		Location	

Description	

When		Doctor	
Condition		Location	

Description	

When		Doctor	
Condition		Location	

Description	

When		Doctor	
Condition		Location	
Description			

When		Doctor	
Condition		Location	
Description			

When		Doctor	
Condition		Location	
Description			

When		Doctor	
Condition		Location	
Description			

When		Doctor	
Condition		Location	

Description	

When		Doctor	
Condition		Location	
Description			

When		Doctor	
Condition		Location	
Description			

When		Doctor	
Condition		Location	
Description			

When		Doctor	
Condition		Location	
Description			

Hospital Packing List

Clothing	

Toiletries	

Technology	
Phone & Charger	

Food & Drink	
Water Bottle	

Medical Items	
Healthcare meets Selfcare	
Medication	
Relevant Documents & Cards	

Selfcare & Other Items	
Eye-mask & Ear plugs	

We are so proud of you!

We're sorry if it's been a tough time, know that you don't deserve to be putting up with all of this. We hope that, even if it was only a little, this book helped you with your medical journey; Not only for self-care, but for clear communication with your health-care team. If this book was useful, feel free to check out the rest of the Health-Care meets Self-Care collection & purchase The Chronic Illness Tracker. To provide any feedback, feel free to email takecarewithlana@gmail.com.

Wish you all the best!